THE MOLD CURE

Natural and Effective Solutions to Mold Growth, Allergies, and Mycotoxins

By Joey Lott

www.joeylotthealth.com

Publishing services provided by **Archangel Ink**

ISBN: 1518666310
ISBN-13: 978-1518666315

Table of Contents

My Introduction to Mold..5

What is Mold? 13

Mycotoxins 16

You're Not Crazy...21

How to Know if You Have a Mold Problem...............23

Reducing Moisture...28

Cleaning 38

Carpets and Mattresses 44

Essential Oils...50

Air Filters...59

Reducing Mycotoxin Load 64

4

Get to It 74

Get My Future Books FREE 77

Connect with Me 78

One Small Favor 79

About the Author 81

My Introduction to Mold

In 2006, I moved from sunny Southern California to New England. The humidity, reminiscent of my childhood in the suburbs of St. Louis, felt oppressive-- my clothes would be drenched with sweat during the muggy summer days. And within the first several weeks in my new apartment, the basement flooded *three* times. New England has a *lot* of water compared with places like Southern California or New Mexico, and water, as we'll see, means mold growth.

Before I moved to New England, I had progressive health problems including the results of years of restrictive eating disorders, extreme anxiety, obsession, compulsion, and paranoia (all of which may have potentially made me for vulnerable to mold allergies), but I still had energy. Yet when I moved to New England, my energy levels dropped dramatically. While I lived in Southern California, I had been a *fanatical* yoga practitioner, doing an hour or two of often intense practice every day. But within a few months of being in

New England, I found that I didn't have the energy to practice any longer.

In 2010, after contracting Lyme disease, I moved with my partner into a small cabin in the hills of southern New Hampshire where it rains or snows half the days of the year. After a particularly damp and unseasonably warm winter, we began to notice mold growing on the wall. After a few months of deteriorating health, we moved into another, nearby cabin. Being set back in the woods with little sunlight and being insulated with straw bales, this cabin too was moldy, but only mildly, and despite my ongoing health problems, I felt a tremendous relief in the new environment.

In the new cabin, I began a journey toward improved health and well-being. After trying an exhausting number of things in hopes of healing, including an unbelievable number of different herbs, vitamins, minerals, and supplements of all sorts along with shiatsu, homeopathy, qi gong, and plenty of other things done in desperationI finally discovered the essential and remarkably simple things that helped me to rediscover health. Among the key components were eating *way* more food in an unrestricted fashion, discovering effective ways to release chronic stress patterns, and correcting a long-term habit of chronic hyperventilation--all things I have written about in other books.

So it was that I began to feel much better. In fact, leaps and bounds better. Some months after I had made a remarkable recovery, my partner, our children, and I (along with our dog) embarked on an adventure, driving west and settling in New Mexico where we lived for a year. During that time, my health continued to improve. I felt stronger and more energetic with each day.

Though we loved New Mexico, we made the decision to move back to New Hampshire again to live in the community where we had previously lived; to be among friends and a large number of children for our children to have those important connections. We packed up the car and headed east.

The town where we live is tiny with less than a thousand inhabitants. So rental housing doesn't come available with great frequency. However, we were fortunate enough to find a house for rent not only in the town, but within a relatively short distance from our friends. So we snatched up the opportunity and signed a lease despite my reservations about the mold.

When I had visited to look at the house, I smelled the mold immediately. And, after being in the house for half an hour, my eyes were burning, my nose was running, and I felt generally lousy. Still, it was the *only* place available, and so we took it. Even though I knew that mold and I had a strained relationship, to put it mildly, I hoped that my improved health would allow me to function well despite the mold. I purchased a high-capacity dehumidifier and pump to place in the basement, which was *by far* the moldiest place in the house, hoping that would resolve most, if not all of the excess mold.

Immediately after moving in, I felt bad. My eyes were irritated and glossy, I felt extremely fatigued, and my muscles contracted involuntarily. But the most intense aspects of the experience were the neurological symptoms, which are best summed up as "brain fog." It was as though my brain wasn't working well. I felt cognitively oppressed, as though a heavy, thick fog had descended upon my head. I felt easily irritated; whereas I normally had nearly unending patience with my kids, suddenly I felt so uncomfortable that when they weren't doing things the way I wanted (which, let's face it, is most of the time), I felt a sense of urgency as though something needed to be resolved.

Of course, we immediately began cleaning the place, hoping that would help. But after helping my partner move a dusty piece of furniture (one that came with the house) one morning, I became almost completely disabled. The experience is difficult to describe to someone who has never experienced it, but although I felt that I had the physical capacity to do things, suddenly I was incapable of mustering the will to do anything. This was a *very* familiar feeling--one I had experienced for many months while we lived in the first moldy cabin.

My children also began exhibiting strange behavior. My daughter particularly took a major turn for the worse in that she became much more irritable and began complaining of aches and pains in her joints. Her sleep became fitful and disturbed, and she developed bags under her eyes. Her behavior reminded us of how she used to be before we had moved to New Mexico. The improvement in New Mexico was something we had chalked up to "growing out of a phase", but upon reflection, it now seems more likely that mold allergies may have accounted for much of the difficult behavior she had exhibited when we had previously lived in New Hampshire.

I began to research for effective, natural solutions to mold overgrowth and the resultant symptoms that can occur in humans. What I found was that the books that I came across generally failed to provide a comprehensive, well-researched, honest view of the situation. I did come across one excellent book called *The Mold Survival Guide* written by Jeffrey and Connie May. That book is a wealth of information written by a home inspector and a microbiologist that details how to successfully remediate mold in a building. However, it didn't give any information about how to address the health effects of mold exposure. Other books that I found that did address the health effects tended to fall short of my expectations. Namely, I wanted well-researched information about how to safely and naturally remediate mold problems and address health complications related to mold exposure. I wanted something that I could do myself (i.e. no expensive consultations, tests, or prescription drugs) and that I could have confidence that it would work.

Furthermore, as I began to look through the internet for information, I came across no shortage of poorly researched and dangerous advice being given by those in pursuit of solving their perceived mold problems. Often there would be no emphasis on removing the sources of mold growth nor the actual toxins that can cause symptoms. Instead, there were often instructions to "bathe in ammonia" or take a variety of supplements that, when I researched them, had absolutely no evidence to support the idea that they could possibly help reduce the toxic load from mold mycotoxins while some of them could be toxic themselves!

Eventually, after sifting through countless scientific and medical publications and abstracts and reviewing reputable literature regarding how and why mold grows and how mold can produce symptoms in humans, I had some solid information. Putting what I learned into practice helped tremendously.

In this book, my intention is to share with you the fruits of my research and experience. I will share with you some of the basics of how and why mold grows and the most effective ways in which you can reduce mold growth in your home. I will also share with you how mold can affect human health and how you can reduce the toxins produced by mold as well as reduce the negative effects on your body.

Everything that I share with you in this book is free of harmful synthetic chemicals such as fungicides and antifungal pharmaceuticals, and it is also effective. With that said, it's not all cheap. The fact of the matter is, once you've got a mold problem, dealing with it effectively will require a financial investment. However, unlike other publications on the subject of mold remediation and health restoration, I make every effort to suggest the most cost efficient way in which to successfully reduce mold and toxins while bolstering your health. I am sensitive to the financial considerations of how to successfully improve conditions without breaking the bank. Yet if you truly want to make positive and sustainable changes when it comes to mold, you'll be best off doing it right from the beginning, which may require some upfront costs of hundreds of dollars (or euros or pounds or whatever may be the case).

And finally, before moving on, I want to tell you that sometimes the only feasible solution short of a complete, professional mold remediation (which often means removing and replacing large amounts of building materials) is to move. In my own case that is what we finally decided to do. Although the changes that I was able to make proved very helpful, in the end they weren't sufficient. In our case we were dealing with a 200 year old house with a basement composed of a soil floor and sweating rock walls, an attached barn, an attic used as storage for the landlord's moldy possessions, and a badly insulated roof that produced condensation on the rafters. The house itself is situated with woods encroaching to the west and a thick sugarbush to the east, meaning that at no point in the day does the house receive adequate sunlight. Add to that poor drainage and the fact that the landlord had sealed up the basement, providing perfect conditoins for mold growth. Finally, we had to conclude that the necessary financial investment to sufficiently reduce the mold in the house was beyond our means, especially as renters. And although we were all feeling better with the steps I took, my daughter was still having fitful sleep, inflammation in the joints, and frequent bouts of extreme irritability. We made the decision to move. And given similar circumstances I would advise anyone who can to move as well. So keep that in mind as you read this book. If you can catch a mold problem in time and/or if the problem is small and isolated, the remedies in this book should prove very useful and effective. But there are always limits. So use good judgment.

What is Mold?

Unfortunately, many people are poorly informed about what mold is and isn't, and understanding the nature of mold really is an important first step in this process. A clear understanding of what mold is and what it does can provide a platform for effectively dealing with any mold problems.

Mold refers to a class of fungi containing tens or hundreds of thousands of different species, depending on which expert you consult. Regardless of the specific number of species, there are lots, and there are *lots* of individual mold organisms of each type of species.

Mold is ubiquitous, meaning that it is everywhere. So before we even get started talking about how to remediate mold problems, it is important that you understand that it is completely unrealistic to completely eliminate mold. And that is okay. Small amounts of mold are fine. It's just large amounts of mold growth that are problematic, and we'll be looking at ways to reduce the amount of mold in your home environment.

Mold, being fungi, are not plant, animal, bacteria, algae, nor virus. They *are*, however, more closely related to other fungi such as mushrooms and yeast. Like other fungi, molds are powerful and important decomposers. They play crucial roles in environmental health; by "digesting" organic matter (such as plants and animals), they help to recycle nutrients, making them available for other organisms.

However, when found in large concentrations, mold can pose a hazard to human (and other animal) health. Mold reproduces by creating and dispersing large numbers of tiny (microscopic) spores, which are capable of creating new clones of the mold. Large numbers of spores can cause allergic reactions in animals, including humans.

Molds also produce substances known as microbial volatile organic compounds (MVOCs), which also cause health problems when found in sufficient quantities. According to the Environmental Protection Agency (EPA), MVOCs are linked with "headaches, nasal irritation, dizziness, fatigue, and nausea," though every piece of literature I have found on the subject admits that MVOCs are poorly documented and poorly understood to date. So other symptoms may be associated with them. In any case, MVOCs are what cause mold to have a smell. When you walk into a musty or moldy-smelling area, what you are smelling are MVOCs rather than the mold itself.

Many researchers believe that the presence of large concentrations of spores and MVOCs are the primary cause of symptoms[1]. However, it is also clear that at least some symptoms associated with mold are due to the presence of *mycotoxins*, which are substances that molds produce in order defend themselves and their food from other organisms such as bacteria. There are a tremendous number of mycotoxins, and they are not all well understood, but it is quite obvious that they can produce unpleasant and sometimes lethal effects on humans and other animals--a matter we'll look at in more detail in the next section. In *most* cases mycotoxins probably play a relatively small role in mold-related symptoms. However, that doesn't mean they should be dismissed entirely as potential causes of symptoms.

Some individuals may potentially develop lung infections due to inhaling mold spores, though it is not extremely likely. It's also worth mentioning that although it is thought to be rare, it *is* possible for mold to infect humans *systemically*. Generally, systemic mold infections are believed to occur only in people with severely compromised immune systems.

In summary, if you have a mold problem, then you've got several things that you've got to address. First, you've got to reduce the factors contributing to growth, which is mostly moisture, as we'll see. That will halt the growth, but you'll still have spores, MVOCs, and mycotoxins hanging around, which you'll need to deal with. We'll see how to do that later in the book.

---

[1] Edmondson et al. Allergy and "toxic mold syndrome". Annals of Allergy, Asthma, & Immunology. 2005; 94(2): 234-239.

Mycotoxins

Many books and online resources regarding mold sensationalize mycotoxins, pointing out that they have been used as biological warfare agents. On the other hand, many conservative agencies such as the EPA or the Centers for Disease Control (CDC) downplay the potential for harm when it comes to *environmental* exposure to mycotoxins. I suspect that the truth is somewhere in between. Mycotoxins are often extremely strong substances that have profound effects on other living organisms, including humans, and large concentrations of them are likely very bad for health. But I don't believe it is useful to be alarmist about it either since the truth is that there just isn't a great deal of good research yet into how mycotoxin exposure in indoor environments really affects humans.

There are a lot of different types of mycotoxins, and not many of them are yet known. Some of them, however, are already extremely well known. Perhaps the most famous mycotoxin is known as the antibiotic drug penicillin, which is produced by *Penicillium* mold. In fact, penicillin was first discovered because it was noticed that nothing would grow near *Penicillium* mold, hence the name of the drug, antibiotic, meaning "against life."

Like penicillin, most mycotoxins seem to serve the function of defending a fungus's territory. And, like penicillin, other mycotoxins are, as the name suggests, toxic in sufficient amounts. Some other mycotoxins are as *in*famous as they are famous. One such example are the mycotoxins produced by ergot, which is a fungus that grows on many grains. The ergot mycotoxins are responsible for what is known as ergotism, a condition that can produce gangrene and convulsions. (Though, it is worth noting, like penicillin, ergot mycotoxins in controlled doses and/or when further modified have proven to be valuable medicines.)

Yet another infamous mycotoxin is a substance (or, rather, a class of substances) known as aflatoxin. Aflatoxin is produced by *Aspergillus* molds, which are ubiquitous, and it came to fame after an incident in the 1960s in which approximately 100,000 young turkeys died in England. The condition was known as Turkey X disease, and it was later found that it had been caused by aflatoxin contamination of the turkey feed.

Aflatoxin is extremely carcinogenic. In fact, it is used in laboratories in order to produce cancer in animals (the ethics of which are, of course, questionable, to say the least), which it does reliably. Not only does aflatoxin produce cancer, however, it can also be acutely lethal in large enough doses. For example, as recently as 2004, a significant event of aflatoxin poisoning killed 125 Kenyans, and it was found that their corn was contaminated with mold. In the U.S. in the 1990s, aflatoxin outbreaks were found to be caused by contaminated peanut butter. And aflatoxin contamination kills or harms countless animals each year due to contaminated feed.

Clearly, to date, the most significant mycotoxin outbreaks have been associated with *eating* contaminated foods. However, that does not mean that significant exposure through other routes, such as inhalation, may not also pose serious health risks. Thus far no studies confirm a causative link between inhalation of mycotoxin and any specific disease states. However, some studies to show a link. For example, a study of livestock feed processing company employees[2] (who are subject to a large amount of aflatoxin dust) showed no increased risk of lung cancer but did show an increased risk of liver cancer. Other studies[3] suggest that inhaled aflatoxin may potentially be linked to lung cancer. Italian doctors published a case study of a woman who developed acute kidney failure after inhaling mycotoxins in a granary[4]. On the other hand, a team of toxicologists modeled what they believed to be the maximum amount

---

[2] Olsen et al. Cancer risk and occupational exposure to aflatoxins in Denmark. British Journal of Cancer. 1988; 58(3): 392-396.

[3] Kelly et al. Aflatoxin B1 activation in human lung. Toxicology and Applied Pharmacology. 1997; 144(1): 88-95.
and

Viegas et al. Occupational exposure to aflatoxin (AFB_1) in poultry production. Journal of Toxicology and Environmental Health. 2012; 75(22-23): 1330-1340.

[4] Di Paolo et al. Inhaled mycotoxins lead to acute renal failure. Nephrology Dialysis Transplantation. 1994; 9 Supplement 4: 116-120.

of mycotoxins that could be inhaled in 24 hours at the highest levels reported for a bunch of mycotoxins in indoor environments and concluded that that level of mycotoxins isn't likely to pose a health risk[5]. Several other studies draw similar conclusions, though they also admit that the truth simply isn't yet known.

So, while there isn't enough evidence to be alarmist about exposure to indoor mycotoxins, there is reason to be *cautious* when it comes to them. I believe that many so-called mold "experts" are preying on people's fears and over-hyping the mycotoxin risk. However, there simply hasn't yet been enough good research into the actual risks involved in inhaling mycotoxins and otherwise being in a moldy indoor environment to write off the risk. It is entirely possible that the toxicologists who modeled indoor mycotoxin inhalation failed to account for some factors that could influence the actual amount of mycotoxins likely to be present. It is also possible that they aren't accounting for other routes of exposure. For example, moldy homes may result in more mold and mycotoxins on food, which may produce a larger exposure than inhalation alone. Furthermore, mycotoxins inhaled may be filtered back up into the throat by way of tiny hairs called cilia that line the bronchi, at which point the mycotoxins may be swallowed. While these latter points are somewhat speculative, the point is that there is no final word on this matter just yet. And until then, it is sensible to be prudent but not afraid.

---

[5] Kelman et al. Risk from inhaled mycotoxins in indoor office and residential environments. International Journal of Toxicology. 2004; 23(1): 3-10.

You're Not Crazy

If you suspect that you have mold growth or the conditions for mold growth in your home then it is very prudent to take steps to eliminate mold growth. However, some people will poo-poo the idea, suggesting that you're over-reacting and that "a little mold never hurt anyone". While it's true that becoming obsessive about mold is unhealthy, it's also true that mold growth for those who are sensitive really does produce genuine health consequences. As such, taking reasonable steps to reduce mold growth is a very good idea. If you are sensitive to mold or if anyone in your home is a child, pregnant, elderly, or chronically ill then reducing mold growth becomes even more important.

A number of studies have demonstrated the very real consequences of mold exposure. Not everyone reacts to mold, which is why some people have an extremely casual attitude toward it. However, a significant percentage of people do. In study conducted by the Medical College of Wisconsin which I referenced earlier, the researchers found that in addition to the typical symptoms associated with allergies such as runny nose, headache, and cough, mold-exposed participants also experienced fatigue (23 percent) and nervous system symptoms (25 percent). Researchers from the U.S. Veterans Affairs have also concluded that mold exposure produces a variety of symptoms beyond classic allergic responses, including cognitive deficits and increases in depression[6].

How it is that people become sensitized to mold is still not well understood. It is generally accepted that children, pregnant women, elderly people, and people with chronic illness or compromised immunity are at the greatest risk. However, there may be other factors that aren't yet understood. In any case, it does seem that the greater and longer the exposure to mold, the greater the likelihood of developing mold sensitivities. Therefore, reducing mold growth is *always* advisable, even if the occupants of a home do not yet show any mold sensitivities.

---

[6] Baldo et al. Neuropsychological performance of patients following mold exposure. Applied Neuropsychology. 2002; 9(4): 193-202.

How to Know if You Have a Mold Problem

Determining *if* you have a mold problem is a logical first step in the process. If you do not have a problem, then trying to solve that problem obviously won't yield positive results. For example, if you are sick with, say, a bacterial infection, trying to fix a non-existent mold problem won't be helpful; it would just be expensive.

So how can you know if you have a mold problem? Probably the most effective way to get a strongly conclusive (though obviously not infallible) answer to whether you have mold problems or not is to hire a professional mold inspector to come and do an inspection. Unfortunately, this is also generally expensive with reported costs anywhere from 300 USD to more than ten times that much! Reportedly, some mold inspectors will do free inspections, but I haven't found any in my area, and if you find such an offer, make sure that you read the fine print. The benefit of professional inspection is that mold inspectors know where to look, what to look for, *and* they generally have some expensive gadgets such as laser particle counters that help to find mold that can't be seen. But the cost is often prohibitive if you have to pay.

If you choose *not* to have an inspection done (I did not, for example), then you can at least do your own inspection. Obviously, most of us won't have the aid of thermal imaging devices or laser particle devices to help us. So instead, we've got to search based on our senses. An unaided mold inspection will rely on the senses of sight, smell, and touch. You'll also want to use some deductive reasoning to find the most likely places for mold, which will generally be cool, damp, and/or dark.

In order to use your sight to detect mold, you'll be looking for mold growth, not spores. That's because mold spores are microscopic, and it's not until they begin to form colonies that you can see them. You're probably accustomed to seeing mold growing on bread or fruit. That type of mold is often green or sometimes white or grey in appearance, and it can seem hairy. Other types of mold are darker green or even black. Most of the time you'll see mold growing in circular patches, though depending on what the mold is growing on and how long it has been growing, you may find patches of mold that are shaped in non-circular patterns. You may see mold growing in all kinds of locations including walls, ceilings, floors, cabinets, shelves, closets, books, curtains, beds, clothing, and just about anything that either is made of organic (plant or animal) material or that is coated in organic material (i.e. dust). When we started looking, we found mold growing even on glass because the glass had an extremely thin layer of dust on it.

Not *everything* that looks like mold is actually mold, however. There are other things that can appear like mold, including something called efflorescence, which is a crystalline growth formed by minerals, and it is harmless to health. Efflorescence only appears on concrete, brick, or stone.

Reportedly, some people also mistake soot for mold. So if you find what you suspect may be black mold, you may want to check if it is near a flame source such as a fireplace, a candle, or a kerosene lamp.

If you find what you suspect may be mold, but you are uncertain, then you may want to use a UV-A light, commonly known as a black light, to provide some confirmation. If you have a black light that you purchased as a novelty product, then it will probably work for this purpose. However, an LED flashlight that emits light in the UV-A spectrum will probably be better because it is more portable and easier to focus. You can find such flashlights for sale online for approximately 10 to 15 USD. Many lights sold for detection purposes (they are often marketed for detecting animal urine) are at the 395 nm wavelength, which will work for detecting mold. Shine such a light on the suspected mold, and if it fluoresces a green or yellow color, it is likely mold. Plenty of other things will fluoresce, including urine and some household cleaning chemicals, so fluorescence isn't a guarantee of mold, but it can help confirm suspected mold, and it may reveal other mold that wasn't easily detected.

Your sense of smell can be extremely helpful in detecting mold that is actively growing as well. Musty or moldy smells are a *very* strong indicator of mold since growing mold produces an abundance of MVOCs that produce characteristic odors. That doesn't mean that *all* similar smells are indicators of mold since other organisms can produce similar MVOCs. However, generally, musty and moldy smells mean mold.

Not all mold can be seen easily because it may be hiding. Mold prefers dark, damp, cool places. So mold will often grow in places that are out of sight such as behind drywall. If you have reason to suspect mold, and particularly if you can smell mold, you will want to identify cool, damp areas. As we'll see later, areas that can attract mold growth may include roofs, the interiors of walls, and poorly insulated areas of otherwise tightly-insulated structures. That's because they allow water to condense, providing the dampness that mold loves. Mold inspectors may use thermal imaging devices to locate cool areas, but you may just have to use your sense of touch. Alternatively, you may want to invest in an infrared thermometer, which usually start around 17 USD. An infrared thermometer will give you readings of surface temperatures (versus air temperature), which can help you to locate cool spots on walls, floors, ceilings, etc.

And lastly, since mold loves moisture, you should use deductive reasoning to locate any and all places where moisture is likely to be collecting. That may be from condensation, from leaks, or from any other source. Also, appliances with cooling systems such as air conditioners and refrigerators have condensers that can grow mold when dusty due to the damp nature of the component. These appliances may also have drip trays that can also grow mold. Therefore, it is advisable to check these appliances for mold.

Once you have found mold, do *not* begin cleaning. Improper cleaning can stir up lots of spores and mycotoxins, and any allergic reactions will be *much* worse. The first step is simply to identify the locations of the mold. Next, you'll need to change the conditions that have been conducive to mold growth, which we'll explore in the next section.

Reducing Moisture

Once you've found mold, you're ready to start getting rid of it. However, before you do anything else, you're going to want to reduce the amount of moisture. That's because, as I stated earlier, you will *never* get rid of all the mold, but you can reduce the amount and remove the conditions that favor mold growth. If you simply remove the mold to the best of your ability but the moisture is still present, then whatever mold remains (and plenty will, no matter how thoroughly you think you can get rid of it) will continue to grow until you reduce the moisture.

Moisture can appear for many reasons, and so you need to address the underlying cause of the moisture. If there is a leak in the roof, for instance, you will need to repair the leak. If there is a leak in the plumbing, then you will need to repair that. But most often, the moisture is present simply because there is either too much humidity or there are surfaces that are unusually cool or both.

Moisture is going to behave slightly differently depending on the temperatures inside and outside. If the temperature outside is warm or hot (i.e. summer in temperate climates), then the most likely problem is going to be high humidity inside. On the other hand, when it is cold outside and warm inside (i.e. winter in temperate climates), the humidity levels both inside and outside generally are lower, but condensation problems are more likely because of something called the dew point, which we'll explore shortly. First, let's look at the summertime scenarios.

Although, as we'll see shortly, relative humidity isn't always the best way to judge mold growth potential, it is a useful general gauge that is a fairly standard way to measure the amount of moisture in the air. As a rule of thumb, many experts suggest keeping relative humidity levels below 50 percent in order to minimize mold growth. Certainly, if you have existing mold problems, you'll want to reduce the relative humidity to somewhere in the 30 to 50 percent range, which should be comfortable for you but too dry for mold. Does that mean that humidity above 50 percent will *always* result in troublesome mold growth? Obviously not. But in *your* case it has, and so if the relative humidity in your living space (or anywhere in your building) is higher than 50 percent and you have mold growth, reduce the humidity. As we'll see later, simply reducing the relative humidity won't necessarily solve all the moisture problems, but it's a good start and the simplest place to get started.

In some cases, the humidity outside of a home is low enough that it would not support mold growth inside a home, but because the home has poor air exchange rates and normal amounts of moisture are added inside (cooking, showering, etc), the inside humidity is high. In these cases, one possible solution is to improve air exchange. In other words, open the windows and get a fan. In the right environments, that can be all that is necessary.

Another relatively easy fix is when excessive moisture is added inside while outside humidity is low. In that case, reducing the amount of moisture added to the indoor air and/or increasing ventilation will help. Bathrooms, kitchens, and laundry areas are notorious for producing excess moisture. Good ventilation in these areas can help tremendously. Also, make sure that anything that can vent outside does. For example, some clothes dryers can vent indoors, which adds a lot of moisture to the air. Instead, vent clothes dryers outside. Even most apartment clothes dryers have the option of venting through a window, which is better than venting inside.

The preceding two scenarios assume that the outside humidity is low enough that it won't be conducive to mold growth inside. Therefore, by increasing air exchange and reducing moisture added from the inside it is possible to normalize the humidity so that it is the same inside and out. However, merely increasing air exchange will do very little good in reducing existing mold when the outside humidity is high enough. And for many geographic locations, outside humidity is often quite high. So what do you do in that case?

The simple answer is that you need to reduce the amount of moisture in the air inside the home. If the moisture problem *only* occurs when it is hot and the moisture problem is *only* in the living space (i.e. not in an uninhabited basement or attic) then an air conditioner may solve the problem. That's because air conditioners remove moisture from the air. If you use an air conditioner to reduce humidity, you'll need to make sure that it removes the moisture to *outside* the home. Also, if you use a whole house air conditioning system you'll need to keep the vents clean. And if you use a window or wall unit, you'll need to keep the unit clean as well. Vents or machines that aren't kept free of excess dust can breed mold growth.

For all other moisture problems, I strongly recommend using a quality dehumidifier that is appropriate for the amount of moisture that needs to be removed. The higher the humidity and the larger the space, the higher the capacity of the dehumidifier that will be necessary. Most reviews of many dehumidifiers available in big box stores are unfavorable, suggesting that when it comes to mold, they are rarely up to the task. What you should look for is a dehumidifier that can run continuously and has an appropriate capacity given the space and the amount of moisture that needs to be removed.

There are a *lot* of dehumidifiers to choose from, so you'll want to find one that will meet your needs. Conventional advice for selecting an appropriate dehumidifier suggests that you need to determine the cubic feet per minute that you need to dehumidify (which uses a process involving measuring relative humidity and cubic space and using an equation to determine the value). However, I have been advised by a dehumidifier consultant that cubic foot per minute ratings are now obsolete; apparently they only applied to dehumidifiers made using freon, a coolant no longer used.

Reportedly, the most reliable way in which to determine which dehumidifier is appropriate is to consult the coverage area reported for a product. Unfortunately, most manufacturers report coverage areas that are well beyond the actual capacities of the machines. So in order to get a good sense of what a dehumidifier's actual coverage may be, you'll want to consult a third party. There may be other organizations that have independently tested various dehumidifiers, but the one that I know of is a retailer called Allergy Buyer's Club. You can find a chart published by this organization   here: http://www.allergybuyersclub.com/dehumidifier-technical-comparison-chart.html[7].

You can see from the chart that the price points on some of the high-end dehumidifiers are well over 1,000 USD. However, there are a few selections in the 200-300 USD range that are up to the job of dehumidifying spaces up to near 1500 square feet. If you have a mold problem and simply increasing the air exchange and/or reducing the moisture added inside won't solve the problem (i.e. the humidity outside is high), then a

---

[7] I have no affiliation with Allergy Buyers Club. However, this particular chart is very helpful.

dehumidifier is *essential* as far as I can tell. I really cannot see a better, less expensive option. Remember, no matter what else you do, if the moisture remains, the mold will grow back.

Next, you will want to consider a few other things before making a dehumidifier purchase. The first dehumidifier I purchased was intended to run full time in an unfinished basement without a drain in the floor. Therefore, I wasn't particularly concerned about the noise level, but I *did* care about making sure that I wouldn't have to go into the (moldy) basement several times a day to empty the water that had been collected. So I wanted to get a dehumidifier that had a continuous drain option. Normal continuous drain functions rely on gravity, meaning that the drain must be lower than the dehumidifier. Since I needed to drain the water to a level above the dehumidifier (out a ground level window), I needed a pump as well. I chose a model with a built-in pump for the task, but it is also possible to purchase a separate pump and use that with any model that has a continuous drain function.

The other consideration is noise. The second dehumidifier that I purchased was intended for use in our living space. Therefore, I wanted to make sure that it was going to be quiet enough for that purpose. Unfortunately, there is no standard noise level specification for dehumidifiers, so you have to judge by reviews. Again, I find the "expert" reviews at Allergy Buyers Club to be helpful in this regard. I also wanted the convenience of continuous drain for the dehumidifier in the living space, but since I had more drain options in the living space, I opted for a standard continuous drain model without an added pump.

One thing to note regarding dehumidifiers is that they produce heat in order to draw moisture from the air. The heat is a requirement of thermodynamics, so there's no way around it (without defying contemporary scientific theories). As a rule of thumb, assume that a dehumidifier running continuously will probably increase the temperature by 5 degrees F. If you need year-round dehumidification then you may want to use a dehumidifier only during the cooler months while using an air conditioner during the warmer months.

Again, I suggest that you obtain a dehumidifier (or dehumidifiers) with adequate capacity to dehumidify the space in which you place it. Generally, a product with a greater capacity than necessary will be more cost effective than multiple products with insufficient capacity individually, both in terms of upfront costs and energy use. So whenever possible, select a single dehumidifier capable of dehumidifying each space in which you need to reduce moisture. You may need multiple machines, of course, if you have multiple areas in need of moisture control. For example, the house I rented had a basement, a main living space, and an attic, all of which need to be dehumidified most of the year. So that requires three separate machines, which is costly, but apparently necessary. And it's better than having mold growth.

Thus far we've looked at one of the main causes of moisture problems, which is excessive humidity. And, in many cases, reducing humidity to the 30-50 percent range will help tremendously with mold problems. However, it is only *part* of the equation. In addition, surface temperature can play an important role in mold growth. That's because cool surfaces are likely to gather condensation, which can feed mold.

Relative humidity, which is what we are accustomed to hearing about, is a measure of how much water vapor is contained per unit of air *relative to the total capacity* of the air to hold water. As the temperature rises, the air's capacity to hold water increases. What that means is that at a relative humidity of 50 percent, a unit of air contains much more water at 80 F than it does at 50 F. And, more importantly, the combination of relative humidity and temperature makes it possible to predict the temperature at which water will condense--called the dew point. For example, when the air temperature is 80 F and the relative humidity is 50 percent, the dew point is 60 F. What that means is that condensation will form on any surface with a temperature of 60 F or lower. That's why a glass of cold water "sweats" on a hot day; the surface temperature of the glass is at or below the dew point. So, if your home has an air temperature of 80 F and the relative humidity is 50 percent, the chances of mold growing are low in most cases because not a lot of surfaces will have temperatures at or below 60 F. But it could happen, of course. And, if you've heated your house to 80 F in the winter while it is below freezing outside, at some point within the wall, the temperature will drop to below the dew point, causing water to condense there. And that's a reason why basements are notorious for mold growth; the surface temperature of the walls is usually going to be far below the air temperature, causing condensation.

The dew point is an important consideration in all seasons, but it is particularly important during cold winter months because the warm temperature inside will be above the dew point, but wherever a surface is below the dew point, water will condense. So, for example, if a house is tightly insulated except for a few leaks, those leaks may lead to mold growth on walls or in walls at those spots.

There are a number of ways to locate cool surfaces. Obviously, if you *see* water condensing on a surface, that may be a clue that the surface is below the dew point. You can also use your sense of touch to feel for cool surfaces. And lastly, if you want to measure the temperature of a surface, you can use an infrared thermometer. If you use an infrared thermometer, then you'll want to know the dew point, which you can calculate from the temperature and relative humidity (some "weather station" devices will report this value as well). You can find dew point calculators online such as www.dpcalc.org in order to find the dew point given the temperature and humidity. Then, you can find surfaces with temperatures at or below the dew point. That will tell you areas of likely mold growth.

If you find surfaces at or below the dew point, you'll want to increase the temperature of the surface. Sometimes a surface will be below the dew point simply because it is behind an appliance or furniture that prevents good airflow and thus heating from adequately reaching the surface. In that case, moving the appliance or furniture can help. Alternatively, you can increase air circulation using a fan.

On the other hand, some surfaces may be below the dew point because of problems with insulation or because a seam has come loose. In such cases, fixing the underlying cause is probably the best approach.

Cleaning

Once you've successfully reduced moisture levels, you can next begin to clean and remove existing mold. Do *not* dust and sweep. Do *not* move moldy materials without adequate protection. Doing those things will likely dramatically worsen your symptoms. After I moved a dusty piece of furniture from one room to the next, I became incapacitated for nearly a full day. It felt as though my head was filled with a thick fog that pressed outward in all directions. That could likely have been prevented had I taken some sensible steps in advance.

If you have very strong mold reactions, then you will probably be best off using something to filter the air that you breathe. For most people, the best results will be achieved with a *properly-fitted* N95 (or higher) mask in order to reduce the amount of dust, spores, and other particles inhaled. N95 refers to the standard for particle filtration. In this case, it means that the mask, when properly fitted to seal well against the face, will filter 95 percent of airborne particles. You can find N99 and

N100 masks as well, but they are much pricier, and for most people N95 will be just fine. The key is that it must be properly-fitted, which means that you need the right size for your face and you need to adjust it once on to make sure it is snug against the face. Those of us with beards will find that the masks are inefficient since particles will slip in through the sides where the mask cannot seal against the face. In any case, whether an N95 mask won't work for you or you simply don't want to use one, *something* to filter the particles is better than nothing. A t-shirt or scarf wrapped around the nose and mouth will probably help, though it won't offer filtration as good as an N95 mask.

Next, before you do anything else, I suggest that you remove moldy items as much as possible, including rugs, clothes, books, etc. When you do this, place mold-contaminated items into plastic trash bags before moving them to avoid spreading more mold to other areas.

Non-porous items such as glass jars or metal flatware can grow mold if they are coated with even the finest layer of dust. However, they are generally very easy to clean, and no special cleaning agents are necessary. Use water and a damp cloth to wipe away any mold on non-porous items. Allow them to dry, and they will be fine to keep.

The less mold you keep around, the better. So any porous items that you can part with, do so. However, realistically, most people aren't willing to part with much. So you'll want to know how to clean porous items such as clothes and rugs. Anything that can be washed in a washing machine should be. Use borax, which is a natural mineral sold generally as a "laundry booster" in most grocery, natural food, and big box stores (Mule Team is the usual brand). Borax is very effective in cleaning mold. In fact, one study showed that borax was among the most effective (and the *only* natural) products for cleaning mold on porous building materials[8]. So add half a cup of borax to loads washed with hot water. If you are washing a load with cold water, then mix half a cup of borax in hot water so that it fully dissolves, then add that to the wash. You can also add some essential oils to the mix for further coverage of all possible mold. If you add essential oils, then also add a few drops of a *detergent* to the mix. For laundry, the detergent isn't strictly necessary since the machine generally agitates the wash quite well, which will disperse the essential oils. But a few drops of detergent (not soap) will help the oils to disperse[9]. I'd suggest essential oils of thyme or oregano since they consistently demonstrate some of the greatest efficacy against molds as we'll see in a later section. Other essential oils can also be helpful, as I'll explain later.

Note: While borax is a natural mineral and is generally very safe, it is best to avoid ingesting it since large

---

[8] Menetrez et al. Testing antimicrobial cleaner efficacy on gypsum wallboard contaminated with Stachybotrys chartarum. Environmental Science and Pollution Research International. 2007; 14(7):523-526.

[9] Any detergent will work. For those who want to go as natural as possible, you can use a "natural" detergent. For example, we have used Dr. Bronner's Sal Suds, which is less toxic than many detergents such as Dawn (dish detergent) or Tide (laundry detergent). Just remember that soap (like regular Dr. Bronner's soap) won't work as well for this purpose.

amounts can prove fatal (as can baking soda). Small amounts of borax are actually used in many boron nutritional supplements, so it's only the dose that makes it potentially problematic. However, it is best to keep borax (and baking soda) out of reach of children. Also, borax (like baking soda) is very alkaline, and the alkalinity can irritate the sensitive skin. So when using borax, as is suggested later for washing surfaces, wear waterproof gloves to avoid irritation.

If possible, dry anything washed in a washing machine in a dryer on high heat. If not possible or appropriate (i.e. wool items), then hang dry in full sun as the UV rays of the sunlight will ensure that no mold growth remains.

For porous materials that cannot be washed in a washing machine such as unfinished wood items or books, if you absolutely must keep them, I suggest wiping them with a damp cloth. Use a solution of borax and a few drops of essential oils and a drop or two of detergent mixed in hot water to make a thin paste, wet the cloth, and wipe the surfaces as clean as possible. Then, dry the objects in full sunlight, allowing for good air circulation on all sides.

Now, you're ready to move on to the structure itself. I'd suggest that you clean as much dust as possible. Dust provides a great growth medium for mold, so even if there is no visible mold growth, just assume that dust contains substantial mold. Plus, it likely contains lots of spores and mycotoxins. So cleaning up the dust on the floor, furniture, window sills, and so forth will help to minimize the amount of dust that is stirred up and ultimately inhaled.

In order to clean dust you have two options. One is cheap, the other is more expensive. The cheap option is to use a *damp* cloth to wipe up the dust. Do *not* use a duster or a dry cloth since that will stir up the dust. A damp cloth will remove the dust with minimal airborne particles. Obviously, the damp cloth will add a small amount of moisture to the surface being cleaned, but since you've already reduced the humidity adequately, the amount of moisture is insignificant and will evaporate quickly.

The second, more expensive option, is to use a vacuum. *However*, if you use a vacuum, do *not*, use a standard vacuum since that will merely cause massive amounts of spores to go airborne as they shoot out the vacuum exhaust. Instead, the only way to vacuum is using a HEPA vacuum. HEPA stands for high efficiency particulate air, meaning that the vacuum uses a filter medium to remove particles down to 0.3 microns, which is below the size of spores. Note, however, that many mycotoxins are smaller than 0.3 microns, meaning that HEPA vacuums may not capture them. If you want to use a HEPA vacuum, I would suggest using a *sealed* HEPA vacuum, which means the price point starts at around 250 USD for a decent vacuum. So this isn't for those on a small budget. If you cannot afford a sealed HEPA vacuum, just use a damp cloth, which should work as well, if ever so slightly more work.

Once you've got the dust cleaned up, you're ready to clean all visible mold growth from walls, ceilings, floors, and other parts of the structure. Generally, the very best thing to do is to remove and discard all moldy building materials. However, frankly, most of us are simply not in a position to do that. For example, in the house that I rent, I couldn't remove walls and discard beams and rafters because they were saturated with mold. So understanding that the ideal is to remove the moldy items, when that is not possible the next best thing to do is to clean them with a damp cloth using the same borax and essential oil solution used to clean other porous items. Do *not* use bleach. Although bleach is commonly used for this purpose, it is ineffective in the long run. No reputable organization (including the U.S. EPA, the CDC, and the WHO) recommends using bleach to remove mold on porous surfaces.

Once you have wiped the surfaces clean, let them dry well. Make sure that you are keeping the humidity levels low and run a fan on the surfaces to help them dry well.

Carpets and Mattresses

Carpets and mattresses are great growth mediums for mold, and, unfortunately, due to the expense and inconvenience, we often don't want to get rid of them. This produces a problem for anyone with mold sensitivities.

If you have carpeting in your home and you are sensitive to mold *and* if you have the means and the rights to do so, I'd recommend removing them and replacing them with non-porous (sealed) floors. Obviously, that is a giant project with many financial and health concerns of its own, and it is impractical for most people. So if you *must* keep your carpets, I can make some suggestions for how to clean them. Incidentally, if you *do* decide to have the carpets removed, be sure to find someone to do the job who understands and has a good reputation for following best practices for molding carpet removal to avoid spreading lots of mold to the rest of the space. And research the flooring replacements to ensure that it will be something that you can tolerate. Once mold sensitivities start, reactions to other VOCs as are found in both natural and synthetic (paint, varnish, new material off-gassing, etc) can increase.

I have long disliked carpet. However, the house I rented has a room with wall to wall carpet. Not only that, but *old* (and disgusting) wall to wall carpet. Part of my solution was a simple one: we didn't use that room. (We prefer living in small and open spaces anyway, so not using the room was no inconvenience to us.) However, the fact that it is there means that mold is growing on the other side of the door. So I wanted to do something to clean it. Here's my approach.

First off, do *not* shampoo the carpets. Carpet shampooing will add a ton of moisture to carpets that likely already have massive amounts of mold, and the shampoo will not sufficiently inhibit mold growth. So carpet shampooing is like adding fuel to the fire.

Instead, as always, first and foremost, *reduce the moisture*. Secondly, once the space has been below 50 percent humidity for at least several days, I suggest using a high quality sealed HEPA vacuum (while wearing face protection) with a good carpet attachment. Although this won't remove the mold underneath the carpet (in the padding, which is probably where most if it is), it will help to remove the spores and dust in the carpet and reduce the likelihood of airborne particles during day to day use of the space.

For some people, that will be enough. Continue to vacuum the carpet regularly and keep the humidity levels low. If any liquid is spilled on the carpet, get as much of it up as possible and then run a fan where the liquid spilled (along with the means to keep humidity low) to speed the rate at which it dries.

If you find that you *still* react to the mold in the carpet and you are still unwilling or unable to remove the carpet, then there are a few options you can consider. First, you can try *lowering* the humidity to as low as 30 percent. Lower than that can be uncomfortable, and most dehumidifiers won't go lower than that anyway. With lower humidity, any remaining mold should stop growing. It's really hard to imagine that mold could grow at such a low humidity. However, it won't kill the spores. For the most part, killing the spores that are trapped in the padding shouldn't be necessary. However, if you are still having problems and wish to attempt to do so, I can offer a few suggestions.

First, the least expensive option is to use essential oils and a nebulizer to disperse the essential oils in the room with the carpet. We'll explore this option in more detail in the next section.

A more expensive but possibly more effective approach is to use a true steam cleaner. In fact, a recent study[10] showed that steam cleaning was vastly superior to any other tested method when it came to eliminating mold. In the study, steam cleaning removed between 92 and 99 percent of the mold spores in carpet.

A true steam cleaner is not to be confused with the hot water carpet cleaning machines often marketed as "steam cleaners.". Instead, a true steam cleaner has a boiler that raises the temperature of the water (only

---

[10] Ong et al., Mold Management of Wetted Carpet. Journal of Occupational and Environmental Hygiene. 2014:0.

water is used - no chemicals) to hot enough to produce steam (higher than 212 F or 100 C) and then releases it with pressure (on demand) through a nozzle that you can direct at the surface to be cleaned. High quality (i.e. effective) steam cleaners are generally *expensive*. The Ladybug cleaners, which are among the best available for residential use,) start at 1300 USD, for example. Some less expensive models are available as well. What you want to make sure of when looking for a steam cleaner is that the temperature at the tip of the nozzle is at least 212 F (100 C). Most publish the *tank* temperature, but the temperature at the tip of the nozzle is what is most important.

To clean a carpet with a steam cleaner you will need to use the correct attachment and go over the carpet *slowly* in order to penetrate effectively into the carpet with the steam. Yes, this will add very small amounts of water to the carpet. However, it is fairly insignificant as long as the humidity in the room is low, and as the study showed, this method reduces the spore count impressively -- not just initially, but in the long term.

If your carpet is new or if you have had the carpet cleaned with detergents or chemicals in the past, steam cleaning will release chemicals from the carpet. Therefore, those with chemical sensitivities should not do such a job without proper respiratory protection (a cheap N95 mask will not do) and good ventilation for the room.

The other advantage of steam cleaning is that it will typically make vacuuming more effective, releasing more particles from the carpet. So in the long run, though expensive, steam cleaning in conjunction with dehumidification and HEPA vacuuming seems to be the best option for removing mold from wall to wall carpet.

Mattresses can be treated in the same way as carpets. However, unlike carpets, simply drying and vacuuming probably won't be sufficient for truly sensitive people. That's because the nightly movement (getting on and off, rolling over, etc.) and the close proximity of the nose to the mattress generally means more stuff trapped in the mattress will get release and inhaled. However, mattresses have a significant advantage over carpets in that they can be placed outdoors in the sunlight. UV rays from the sun can kill mold and spores. So I suggest placing the mattress outside on a sunny day. Make sure to elevate the mattress well off the ground to avoid trapping moisture underneath it. Also, to help move trapped contents out, beat the mattress with a suitable device such as a baseball bat [11]. Wear appropriate protective gear to avoid inhaling spores.

Unless you already own or have access to a steam cleaner, purchasing a steam cleaner just to save your mattress may be misguided. But, if you have access to a steam cleaner, then it can be used to clean a mattress just as it can be used to clean a carpet. I would suggest doing it outside on a sunny day with the mattress elevated from the ground (using whatever you would use to sun it). Even though doing it outside will offer good ventilation, using a filtration mask may be a good idea. That is

---

[11] You may also find that this step is more enjoyable if you shout "PC Load Letter" while beating the mattress. And to refresh your memory as to *why* that might make it more enjoyable, watch *Office Space*.

especially true if you are cleaning a conventionally-produced mattress containing flame retardants. Once you've steamed the mattress thoroughly on all sides, dry it well in the sun.

Essential Oils

Essential oils, distilled from plants, are used in a wide variety of applications, both personal and commercially. Many people are familiar with essential oils because they are used for fragrance and for therapeutic properties in personal care products ranging from massage oils to soaps. Some essential oils are used in treating topical fungal infections such as lemongrass for ringworm[12] and tea tree for dandruff, which may be caused by fungus[13]. But commercial industries have been researching essential oils for applications in which antifungal pharmaceuticals and chemical pesticides have been failing due to fungal resistance. And many of those applications are for the reduction of mold and mold mycotoxin production.

---

[12] Kishore et al. Fungitoxicity of essential oils against dermatophytes. Mycoses. 1993; 36(5-6): 211-215.

[13] Nenoff et al. Antifungal activity of the essential oil of Melaleuca alternifolia (tea tree oil) against pathogenic fungi in vitro. Skin Pharmacology. 1996; 9(6): 388-394.

Not a great deal of research has been done into mold remediation in buildings using essential oils. The few studies that I have found that suggest that essential oils can be useful for the purpose merely demonstrate that essential oils are effective against specific molds in test tubes. One, a study from the University of British Columbia[14], demonstrated that the essential oil from cedar leaf is effective against common indoor molds (as well as problematic bacteria). Another from a university in Croatia[15], tested thyme essential oil against samples of indoor molds and concluded that thyme is very effective against them.

When it comes to whether or not essential oils will work to reduce molds in an actual indoor environment and the best means by which to achieve this effect, we are left to rely on anecdotal reports, of which there are *many*.

As stated in the earlier section regarding cleaning, adding essential oils to laundry and to a borax solution for cleaning porous objects and materials can help reduce mold counts. When you add essential oils to a load of laundry, you can add 5 to 20 drops of essential oils directly to the wash for most essential oils. Since the laundry will get a thorough rinsing and then will be dried either in a dryer or by hanging out in the sun, it is

---

[14] Hudson et al. The Antimicrobial Properties of Cedar Leaf (Thuja plicata) Oil; A Safe and Efficient Decontamination Agent for Buildings. International Journal of Environmental Research and Public Health. 2011; 8(12): 4477-4487.

[15] Segvić et al. Antifungal activity of thyme (Thymus vulgaris L.) essential oil and thymol against moulds from damp dwellings. Letters of Applied Microbiology. 2007; 44(1): 36-42.

extremely unlikely that the essential oils would cause any skin irritation when clothes are later worn, but it is possible that incredibly sensitive people may react. So if you or someone in your family is that sensitive, keep that in mind. And I'd suggest that you *not* use cinnamon essential oil for laundry just to avoid the risk of irritation since that is the most likely to cause skin reactions.

For cleaning surfaces with a borax solution and essential oils, I'd suggest that you can probably use about the same number of drops of essential oils in half a cup of thick borax solution as you would use for a load of laundry. Even more would probably be fine. However, make sure that you wear gloves that will keep both the borax and the essential oils off your skin. Most of the essential oils that I recommend in this book won't irritate the skin of most people when diluted. However, some such as cinnamon, can irritate, even when diluted, and people with particularly sensitive skin will be best to avoid touching them. In any case, as stated earlier, concentrated borax with its high pH will irritate the skin anyway, so you will want to use gloves regardless.

It's also worth mentioning that those with extremely sensitive noses may find the smell of essential oils to be overpowering. Therefore, if you or someone you live with has reason to be concerned, either don't use them or at least use good ventilation.

Infants and babies are particularly sensitive to some essential oils. Reasonable amounts of essential oils used in cleaning are unlikely to be a problem, but keep very young children away from essential oil bottles, and keep the room well ventilated after cleaning in order not to overwhelm them with the strong smells.

Also, some essential oils are toxic for some non-human animals, even when they are well tolerated by humans. Cats are particularly sensitive as they metabolize some essential oils differently than we do. Dogs can be sensitive to some. And birds are likely sensitive to many. For dogs and cats, the primary risk is from essential oils applied directly to the skin in significant amounts, so for most cleaning purposes, essential oils are unlikely to pose any risk. However, steer clear of the temptation to apply essential oils directly to pet beds or anything else that a non-human animal is likely to be in close contact with or eat or drink from as that can be harmful and even fatal to them.

In research, a great many essential oils can be effective against many molds. However, I wanted to know which essential oils are the most effective against the most of the common types of indoor molds. In particular I was interested in essential oils that demonstrated near 100 percent effectiveness against Stachybotrys chartarum, Aspergillus niger, Cladosporium cladosporioides, and some of the pathogenic Penicillium molds.

Some essential oils show remarkable effectiveness against nearly all the potentially problematic molds. Still, based on my research, I'd recommend a combination of essential oils to achieve maximum effectiveness. Among the most impressive are caraway, lemon basil, oregano, bay (Pimenta racemosa, not to be confused with bay laurel, which is another plant), thyme, cinnamon (both leaf and and bark of Cinnamomum zeylanicum, which is true cinnamon, though cassia, which is often substituted for cinnamon, is also impressive in this regard), clove, and lemongrass. These are my top picks. Some others such as lavender, eucalyptus, tea tree, and rosemary can pinch hit, but they don't test as strongly as the others.

One study out of the Czech Republic[16] tested 20 essential oils for efficacy against common molds (including everything I was interested in except Penicillium) and found that caraway, lemon basil, oregano, bay, and thyme are all nearly 100 percent effective against those molds. Note that common basil (Ocimum basilicum) did not demonstrate anywhere near the efficacy of lemon basil, so it should not be substituted. Similarly, marjoram (Origanum majorana) did not test as strongly as oregano (which is closely related) and should not be substituted.

The Czech study is not the only one to demonstrate the efficacy of thyme. Many others, including the Croatian study cited earlier have found thyme to be very effective against mold, more so than many other oils tested. The Croatian study also found that an extract of thyme oil called thymol was even more effective than thyme oil itself, suggesting that other plants containing thymol are probably effective. Oregano is another source of thymol, so it is no surprise that oregano often tests strongly against mold.

---

[16] Zabka et al. Antifungal activity and chemical composition of twenty essential oils against significant indoor and outdoor toxigenic and aeroallergenic fungi. Chemosphere. 2014; 112: 443-448.

The tropical plants cinnamon, clove, and lemongrass also show up in study after study as being effective against a variety of molds. In fact, in a study from India[17] testing 75 essential oils against Aspergillus niger, the researchers concluded that the most effective were cinnamon, cassia, clove, and lemongrass.

My suggested essential oil combination would include oregano and/or thyme plus cinnamon leaf, clove, and lemongrass. You could feel free to add others, but I'd include those oils at a minimum if possible. Of course, caraway, lemon basil, and bay could all stand in for thyme or oregano, but thyme or oregano are usually easier to find.

It is important that you only use 100 percent pure essential oils in order to get the benefits. Remember that the actual plant constituents in the oil are what make them effective against mold. Synthetic fragrance oils will not have the same effect. Nor will diluted oils be as effective as pure essential oils. So look for "100 percent pure essential oil" or something of the sort on the label. Oh, and don't get suckered into buying oils from multi-level marketing companies like Young Living Oils and doTerra. They are *way* overpriced and they teach unsafe practices (such as ingesting essential oils, which is *not* a good idea in almost every case). Instead, purchase reasonably-priced, high quality essential oils from reputable companies.

There is one more way to use essential oils that I'd like to share with you. Frankly, I cannot find a single

---

[17] Pawar VC and Thaker VS. In vitro efficacy of 75 essential oils against Aspergillus niger. Mycoses. 2006; 49(4): 316-323.

peer-reviewed study showing the efficacy (or not) of this approach. However, there are lots of anecdotal reports of this working well, and I have used it with some success in spaces where I could not reasonably clean satisfactorily. (For example, the attic of the house I rented is a storage space for the landlord who lives out of the country, so cleaning it adequately was not possible.)

The suggestion is to use a nebulizer in order to diffuse the essential oils as a fine aerosol in the space that you want to disinfect. Specifically, you will want a "jet" nebulizer or "atomizer" which has been tested for use with essential oils. The correct type will require only essential oils be added- - no water- - and it will consist of a small compressor and a glass bulb connected by way of a small tube. The compressor forces air into the bulb which breaks up the essential oils into tiny particles, sending them out of the top of the bulb as a fine aerosol that cannot be seen. They typically are rated for spaces from 150 square feet (small) to 900 square feet. You should look for one with the capacity for the space you want to treat[18].

For most people inhaling the essential oils won't be a problem. In fact, nebulizers are used by "aromatherapists" and essential oil enthusiasts specifically for the purpose of filling an inhabited room

---

[18] The most reasonably-priced and highest quality nebulizer that I have found that is suitable for this purpose is sold by both Mountain Rose Herbs and Star West Botanicals. It is less expensive from Mountain Rose Herbs by a few dollars as of this writing. As a plus, the nebulizer is said to be suitable for up to 900 square feet.

with a fine aerosol of pure essential oils, so it is generally quite safe with most essential oils, including all included in my list of suggestions with the possible exception of cinnamon when used in large quantities. All the same, for the purposes of disinfecting mold contamination, it is better to run the nebulizer when no one is in the space. That way you needn't worry about having a reaction and you can run it for a long time (which you wouldn't want to do if someone is in the space as it would be overwhelming and more likely to be irritating). Oh, and as I mentioned earlier, many essential oils can be potentially toxic to many non-human animals, even if they aren't problematic for humans. So don't expose cats, dogs, birds, fish, rabbits, or anyone else to the essential oil aerosol needlessly.

I suggest that you fill the essential oil reservoir according to the nebulizer instructions with a combination of essential oils according to my recommendations. Turn on the nebulizer and allow to run in a closed space until it has nebulized all the essential oil. Then wait and see. If, after a few days, you still perceive a mold smell, you can run the nebulizer again.

Nebulizing essential oils can be potentially very helpful in some situations, but it should *not* be used as a substitute for keeping moisture levels low. And, whenever possible, it is best to clean objects and surfaces rather than nebulizing essential oils instead. But, as I have mentioned, there are situations in which nebulizing essential oils may be the best practical option. For example, I've told you about the attic that I could not reasonably clean and the carpets that I could not remove. Since I didn't have the luxury of using a steam cleaner on the carpets, nebulizing essential oils (along with a dehumidifier and a HEPA vacuum) is the next best alternative I have come up with.

Like I wrote earlier, I don't have any peer-reviewed papers demonstrating the efficacy of this approach. So to some extent you have to take it on faith that it can work. I do *not* recommend it as a first line of approach. It is merely an adjunct when other, better options are not available to you.

Air Filters

Now we've covered all the basics of remediation. And for most people, that's all that is necessary. However, for other people there may still be health problems associated with mold that need to be addressed. First among the things that we'll look at in this regard is filtering the air.

If you still experience health problems that seem to be linked to mold exposure and your symptoms improve after being away from your home or the place of mold exposure, then it may be that the air quality in that space is poor. It should be that wiping surfaces and vacuuming with a HEPA vacuum will remove most all of the mold and spores except what may remain inside porous building materials. And as long as the humidity is kept low enough, mold won't grow. Obviously, as stated from the beginning, it is impossible to eliminate *all* mold. But as long as the levels are low enough and the humidity is low enough to prevent growth, most people won't experience any problems.

If you are still experiencing problems associated with the space after reducing humidity, fixing leaks, and cleaning thoroughly, then I suggest that before you do anything else, you reinspect and see if you can find any likely culprits.

However, if you cannot find any likely source of the problem that you can address, you may next want to consider an air filtration device.

There are an *incredible* number of air filtration products on the market, ranging from excellent to ineffective to downright dangerous. If you decide to get an air filtration product, I'll offer you some tips for selecting one that will meet your needs.

First things, first, you want to make sure that you select the *type* of filter that can actually work for you and likely *improve* the air quality rather than producing toxicity. You will want to acquire a true HEPA filter at a minimum. HEPA means that it must filter a minimum of 99.97 percent of all particles down to 0.3 microns, which will cover all spores. Anything that is not HEPA won't work to actually filter the air effectively.

Next, you should also look for something that contains a substantial amount of activated carbon since that will help to bind things like mycotoxins that will not be filtered by the HEPA filter since they are too small.

Some filters contain ultraviolet lamps in the UV-C spectrum because light in that spectrum can kill a lot of bacteria, mold, and other microbes. As long as a filter contains *only* a UV-C lamp and the lamp is completely encased so that you cannot see it, then it probably isn't harmful. The lamp *must* be fully encased because light in that spectrum at high enough intensity can damage your eyes if you look at it for long enough. So you don't want that light getting out. Also, although I don't know of any products that contain lamps that use anything other than UV-C, you still want to make sure that is the case if you purchase a filter with UV light because UV-C will *not* produce ozone whereas other UV light will, and ozone is harmful if inhaled in sufficient quantities. But to me, UV-C is not a selling point in an air filter for a simple reason; as far as I know, UV-C is only effective if there is sufficient duration of exposure. In other words, mold moving past the lamp at the rate that is going to happen in an air filter is likely completely useless. So it probably won't hurt anything, but it probably won't help either.

I strongly suggest that you avoid all "ionizing" air "purifiers" or any air filters that include an "ionizer" feature. That is because despite what the manufacturer may claim, as far as I know, *all* ionizer products create ozone. Ozone is a free radical that *can* kill microbes, but in the same way, it will damage your throat, lungs, skin, hair, eyes, and so forth.

And, just to be clear, you should also avoid all air "purifiers" that explicitly produce ozone, including those that create so-called "arans,", which, it turns out, just produce ozone. Some manufacturers will claim that ozone is harmless because it is natural or they will claim that the product only creates "small" amounts of ozone. But if it produces enough ozone to be an effective disinfectant, then it is enough to harm humans, non-human animals, plants, and even rubber and other substances. If it doesn't produce enough to be disinfectant, then it's useless. So in any case, steer very clear of ozone generators.

Although some relatively inexpensive air filters do exist, you should read the reviews of them to see what others' experiences have been with those products. Also, read the fine print carefully and find out how many air changes the product can produce and how much area they can really cover. Don't trust a coverage specification that is not either provided by a reputable third party or at least independently verified by customers.

It is possible that you can find a good quality air filter that will meet your air filtration needs for less for 400 USD, but I kind of doubt it. And if you are sensitive to chemical odors, then ironically, some customers complain of the off-gassing fumes of some air filters in the low price point. For anyone who genuinely needs an air filter, the higher end filters are probably your best bet, and unfortunately, they are pricey. Austin Air makes some excellent, no bells and whistles, plain-jane, HEPA/carbon filters starting at around 500 USD. And for the true air filter aficionado there is the IQAir line, which use what they call *hyper*HEPA, which filters down to 0.003 microns, which is really small -- over a hundred times smaller than standard HEPA. But you'll have to pay for it since the *cheapest* IQAir filter is 900 USD.

Austin Air does have a 30 day money back guarantee for opened items that have been tested. That does *not* cover shipping costs, so if you decided to return the product, you'd be out probably 100 USD. IQAir also allows returns of opened items for up to 60 days, but they also deduct a 15 percent "restocking fee,", so even just *trying* one of the filters isn't cheap.

I wouldn't recommend getting an air filter unless you are reasonably certain that it is likely to help. Still, for some people the right air filter can make a *huge* difference. So it's worth considering as an option...if you can afford it!

Reducing Mycotoxin Load

For the vast majority of people, the main problem they will experience regarding mold is a combination of allergies to spores and reactions to high concentrations of MVOCs. Once the mold, spores, and MVOCs are reduced sufficiently, the symptoms should disappear. Of course, since the allergic reaction is a learned immune response, once sensitized to mold there is an extremely good chance that one will remain sensitive to mold, even in much smaller amounts than used to provoke a reaction. That is one of the reasons why an air filter may sometimes be helpful, because it can reduce the "normal" amounts of mold and spores to an even lower level, making the environment more hospitable for someone with mold sensitivities.

However, some people may continue to experience symptoms even after the mold is gone and the air is filtered. If that happens, there could be many reasons, but in this section we'll explore a few of the likely reasons.

First off, allergies are immune responses, which can involve a lot of physiological stress and inflammation. In fact, a major part of an allergic immune response *is* inflammation. Inflammation is part of how our bodies defend themselves. However, when the inflammation continues unabated for days, weeks, or months, that can produce a lot of stress in the body that may need to be repaired. So we'll look at ways to help and support that process.

One thing that mold allergies can produce is a lack of appetite. If you had a reduced appetite while exposed to mold, then that habit may have reduced your caloric intake. As I have detailed in many of my other books, a reduction in caloric intake produces lowered metabolic rate, lowered thyroid hormone levels, and lowered immunity. So, if for no other reason, if you ate less for more than a day or two, you would have good reason to still feel lousy.

Numerous studies beginning with the Minnesota Starvation Experiment in 1944-1945 have demonstrated that the symptoms of starvation can set in even with modest calorie restrictions. The Biosphere 2 study showed that 2000 calories a day for a prolonged period was enough to produce symptoms of starvation. And the lead researcher in the Minnesota Starvation Experiment, Ancel Keys, stated that the rehabilitation diet needed to be calorie dense and unrestricted for many months. He estimated that 4000 calories a day for perhaps 9 months was necessary after the men in the study ate 1600 calories a day for just 6 months. So eating more food can be an important part of recovery.

The trend in "health" these days is to recommend restrictive diets as part of the cure for everything from fatigue to cancer. And mold-related illness doesn't escape this trend. It is popular for "experts" and amateurs alike to suggest eliminating sugar, gluten, meat, dairy, corn, eggs, grains, fats, and everything else in order to cure whatever ails you. The popular notion is that one should "starve" the suspected pathogens. And because mold is a fungus loosely related to Candida albicans (in the same way that humans are loosely related to chickens), many claim that the best way to "starve" mold is to follow the very same (unproven and unlikely) diet cure often prescribed on the internet (and in person), which is to eliminate all sugars (including fruit) and sometimes even all carbohydrates. Please *do not follow this misguided advice.*

First off, except for those who are extremely immunocompromised (i.e. unmanaged diabetes, untreated AIDS, etc.) a systemic fungal infection is *extremely* unlikely. Therefore, *there is nothing to starve except yourself.* What is *most* likely is that your metabolic rate has slowed and your body is stressed. You probably need to eat more, not less. And, even if there is anything else going on such as a possible, though unlikely, mycotoxicosis, you can't starve mycotoxins since they aren't living. They are chemicals. And the best way to detoxify is to eat enough, sleep enough, and shed stress.

Sleep is the next most important factor. It's so important I've written a whole book on the subject. You need sleep. You probably need more sleep than you think. You can't get well if you don't sleep enough. Sleep more. Sleep during the dark hours of the evening. Aim for at least 8 hours each night of quality sleep. If your sleep is poor, get my book, *Sleep*, and learn some effective ways to improve your sleep. That can reduce inflammation, rebuild tissue, and normalize immunity whereas getting insufficient quality sleep will have the opposite effect.

Next most important is to shed stress. Numerous studies show that chronic stress lowers metabolic rate, decreases immunity, and increases inflammation. Shedding chronic stress has the opposite effect, improving health in every way. If you experience fear, worry, anxiety, or any other type of chronic stress, learn positive ways to release it. I recommend exploring progressive muscle relaxation, which can be very effective. Or, check out my free video training program, www.peacefulpossibility.com, for my unique approach to releasing chronic stress.

As I have mentioned, it is possible, though not likely, that you may have a mycotoxin load in your body. Many "experts" in the field of mold and health overstate the likelihood of a mycotoxin burden, playing on fear, which I think is unconscionable because there simply is no credible evidence to date showing that there is a likelihood of developing a mycotoxin burden living in a moldy home. That doesn't mean that it *can't* happen. It just means that it's not proven nor likely at this point.

With all that said, the possibility does exist of a mycotoxin burden, even if it is a small possibility. As I have already stated, after reducing moisture, mold count, cleaning, and filtering the air, the next best thing you can do is eat, sleep, and shed stress. If you *still* feel bad, then you can do a few more things to support detoxifying *if* you do have a mycotoxin burden. And don't worry, because none of these things is anything like most of what gets called "detoxification" these days. No green smoothies and no enemas are involved.

First off, let's talk about a substance called glutathione, which is a potent antioxidant synthesized in the body that plays a vital role in the removal of all toxic substances. Consider the case of liver damage caused by acetaminophen (Tylenol); it has been known for decades[19] that the damage is caused by the depletion of glutathione and that increasing glutathione protects the liver. Glutathione is important for protecting the liver and the rest of the body from damage done by chemicals of all sorts, including mycotoxins, and glutathione helps to remove these chemicals from the body.

How can you increase glutathione? Many people have tried supplementing with the antioxidant, but it turns out that it is destroyed in the stomach, making oral supplementation potentially ineffective. However, there are other, natural ways to improve glutathione levels.

For one thing, glutathione is synthesized using the amino acids cysteine, glutamine, and glycine, so adequate dietary levels of these amino acids will aid in glutathione synthesis. Cysteine is usually the limiting factor. Reportedly, cysteine is denatured by high heat such as cooking. So the best sources of cysteine are probably

---

[19] Mitchell et al. Acetaminophen-induced hepatic necrosis. IV. Protective role of glutathione. Journal of Pharmacology and Experimental Therapeutics. 1973; 187(1): 211-217.

unheated. The best dietary source of cysteine is egg white, but, let's face it, most of us don't want to eat raw egg whites. I mean, I eat the yolks raw (yeah, there's a tiny risk of salmonella poisoning, so I'm not suggesting you do it), but the whites? No thanks. So the next best options are raw animal organs. Oh, right, you don't want to eat those raw either, do you? (Well, if you do, you can err on the side of caution by eating the organs such as liver only of grass-fed ruminants [(do *not* eat raw pork organs]) and freeze them for two weeks first.) Okay, so since you probably don't want to eat raw egg whites or raw organs, the next best thing is raw dairy. Yeah, there are those who make a stink about how dangerous raw dairy is, and yes, there really is a very small risk, but the actual risks are generally overstated. Raw dairy is delicious when it comes from healthy cows (or goats or sheep) fed grass and allowed on quality pasture. You may be able to find raw milk near you since raw milk sales are allowed in most (though not all) locales when done on the farm.

But, let's say you're dubious about the safety of eating any of those things raw. Okay. I get it. You want to be cautious. I understand. So then what? Well, you could hand over some cash for biologically active *denatured* whey protein powder, which is available from a variety of sellers. Look only for *denatured* whey since that should (hopefully) mean that the cysteine is denatured. The only two that I have seen *any* tests on are Proserum and Immunocal. They are pricey, but they stand a decent chance of increasing glutathione levels.

Once you're supplying your body with adequate protein of the right sorts, there are a few other things you can do to increase glutathione levels. For one thing, you can supplement with some herbs that may increase glutathione, including turmeric, garlic, and milk thistle seed. Unfortunately, little human research has been done to verify that these herbs can increase glutathione levels in real live humans. But there are plenty of studies showing that they *should*. Since these herbs all have a long history of safe use and improving health, there's nothing to lose by trying them.

Turmeric is most commonly available as a powdered culinary herb. You can use the dried, powdered herb or the fresh herb. You can cook with it or mix a small amount of the dried herb in water and drink that several times a day.

Garlic is reportedly most active for increasing glutathione if you chop and crush it and let it sit for 10 minutes *before* you cook with it. Alternatively, you could chop, crush, and wait 10 minutes and then eat it raw, but frankly, that sounds horrible. So I'd suggest cooking with it, which sounds good. The only problem with cooking is that some of the therapeutic compounds in garlic are cysteine-based, meaning that cooking may make the garlic less potent. Most of the garlic supplements are probably ineffective, but steam distilled garlic oil is reportedly effective[20].

For milk thistle seed, you can either grind the seed fresh in a coffee grinder and take 1/4 of a teaspoon of

---

[20] See http://lpi.oregonstate.edu/infocenter/phytochemicals/garlic/ for a detailed write up of why

that with food or mixed in water several times a day or you can find an encapsulated supplement or an extract (tincture) online or in health food stores.

Finally, when it comes to glutathione, rest, relaxation, sleep, and shedding stress will be essential to increasing your levels.

Next, if you are genuinely concerned about mycotoxicosis, you may want to supplement with sequestering substances for a short while. One of the leading "scare" books on the subject of mold health problems recommends using the drug cholestyramine for all people with mold issues (this is called having a hammer and seeing the world as full of nails). Although I think it is a reckless suggestion, apparently it *does* help some (though certainly not all) people. That's because cholestyramine binds with bile salts in the intestine, sequestering toxins so that they can be excreted rather than absorbed.

In the livestock industry, sequestering agents, including cholestyramine, are a big deal because the generally poor conditions and the unhealthy levels of mold in the feed in most commercial operations leads to a heavy toxin (specifically mycotoxin) burden for many animals. So there is a lot of research aimed at investigating the efficacy of various sequestering agents for livestock. Two completely natural and effective sequestering agents are activated charcoal and bentonite clay. These two both are effective in removing mycotoxins from the intestines. Once the liver has successfully removed mycotoxins from the rest of the body with the aid of glutathione, it will transfer them to the intestines in bile. But since the body normally recycles bile, it will normally reabsorb many mycotoxins. That is why short- term supplementation with sequestering agents may be helpful.

You can find activated charcoal supplements in most natural food stores and probably in many pharmacies. You can also find them online. Follow the instructions on the supplement you choose.

For bentonite clay, any clay intended for internal use (some are not, so make sure it is for internal use) will be fine. In general, calcium bentonite is probably better, but sodium bentonite will be fine short- term. If you're hesitant to ingest clay, then let me give you a little bit of background. First off, it's a "special" clay because it is made from volcanic ash, so it's not the same as the clay you might dig up in your back yard. Second, there are records of humans ingesting this type of clay for a long time. Third, NASA funded research in the 1960s to find the best way to prevent bone loss in weightlessness and found that calcium bentonite was the best. So I'm not proposing something that is *really* weird. Just a little weird[21]. If you get powdered bentonite clay, I suggest you start with 1/2 teaspoon mixed in a glass of water or juice and drink that once a day.

Supplementing with calcium bentonite clay long-term may be all right, though there is some evidence that it may lead to lowered levels of some minerals. Supplementing with activated carbon long- term will

---

[21] If you still think I'm nuts, here's an interesting article that confirms that clay really can help remove mycotoxins: http://www.ncbi.nlm.nih.gov/pmc/articles/PMC3654247/

probably lead to malabsorption issues. So my suggestion is that you use these supplements only in the short term -- for a week or two -- while increasing glutathione levels.

Get to It

I've just given you a lot of information. So now what do you do? How best to get started?

First off, it is important that you keep in mind that your specific experience may require more drastic measures than what I have outlined here. In some rare cases, people really do need to abandon everything and just get the heck out of Dodge. But the fear mongers have overhyped that possibility, and for the overwhelming majority of us, that simply isn't necessary. That's because for most of us, *even in the presence of some Stachybotrys chartarum* (the dreaded "black mold"), the primary symptoms are caused by allergies, and the problem can probably be resolved through the steps detailed in this book without shelling out tens of thousands of dollars. But only you can know. Don't stay on a sinking ship. Do what is appropriate for you and your situation, and make use of the information in this book to help you as best as possible.

Assuming that you are planning to "stand your ground,", the first step is to determine the likelihood of the presence of mold. If you can identify mold in your home, the next step is to find out where the water is coming from, because there will definitely be too much water. In some cases, the water is from a structural leak or from a leak in the plumbing, in which case you'll need to fix the leak. Usually, however, the humidity will be the problem. So test the relative humidity of your home, particularly near where you have found mold. Then, take the steps I outlined throughout the book for reducing moisture.

Once you've successfully reduced the moisture levels, you'll want to clean. Please remember to wear protective gear to avoid inhaling large amounts of spores. Then take care to follow the sensible cleaning suggestions I offered in the book. Namely, avoid stirring up spores and dust into the air.

After you've cleaned, then take a rest. Give it a few days or a week to see how you feel. Hopefully you'll notice a significant improvement. In that case, you're all done with the suggestions in the book.

On the other hand, if you're still feeling lousy, next determine the likely cause. Are you feeling bad in your home but feeling well elsewhere? Then chances are there's still mold or spores in your home that you can either clean or filter.

If you just feel lousy all the time and everywhere, then you may need to boost your metabolism, rest more, and shed stress. You can also take some steps to increase natural detoxification with glutathione and sequestering agents such as clay and carbon.

I wish you the best in your endeavor to improve your living condition. May you be happy and healthy.

Get My Future Books FREE

If you enjoyed this book (Hey, if you made it this far it couldn't have been that bad), you'll probably enjoy many of my other books about health and wellness. And you can get all my new releases in health and wellness for free by signing up for my mailing list at www.joeylotthealth.com. It's simple, it's free, and it's totally honest and legitimate. Nothing scammy or spammy or anything else like that (i.e. I won't be trying to sell you The 7 Dirty Underground Top Secret Weird Tricks for Rock Hard Abs or Young Living Oils). It's just about free books for those who appreciate my work, because I appreciate YOU. Simple as that.

Connect with Me

I welcome your questions, comments, and feedback of any kind. Please feel free to email me at joeylott@gmail.com. I am now receiving so many emails that I cannot always reply to every email. I do read them all, and I do my best to reply to as many as possible. For the benefit of others, I may choose to publish my response to your email on my blog or in book format. I will maintain your privacy and anonymity if I choose to publish my response.

One Small Favor

My sincere goal in writing is to share something that may be of value to you. And I endeavor to do so while keeping the costs low for readers. The success of my books and my ability to reach other readers who may benefit from my books depends in large part on having lots of thoughtful, honest reviews written about my work. You would do me a great favor if you would please take a moment to generously write a review of this book at Amazon.com. This will only take a few minutes of your time, and you will be helping me a great deal. I sure would appreciate it.

About the Author

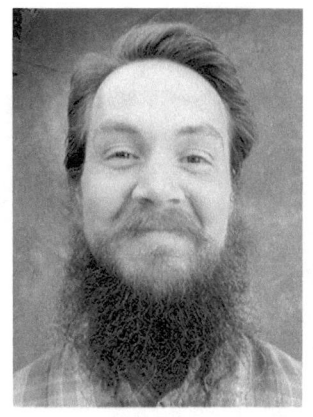

"The secret to happiness is to let go of everything - see through every assumption."

Beginning at a young age Joey Lott experienced intensifying anxiety. For several decades he lived with restrictive eating disorders, obsessions, compulsions, and an inescapable fear. By the time he was 30 years old he was physically sick, emotionally volatile, and mentally obsessed with keeping any and all unwanted thoughts and experiences at bay.

At this time Lott was living on a futon mattress in a tiny cabin in the woods. He was so sick that he could barely move. He was deeply depressed and hopeless. All this despite doing all the "right" things such as years of meditation, yoga, various "perfect" diets, clean air, and pure water.

Just when things were at their most dire, a crack appeared in the conceptual world that had formerly been mistaken for reality. By peering into this crack and underneath all the assumptions that had been unquestioned up to that moment, Lott began a great undoing. The revelation of this undoing is that reality is utterly simple, ever-present, seamless, and indivisible.

Lott's books provide a glimpse into the seamless, simple, and joyous nature of reality, offering a glimpse through the crack in conceptual worlds. Whether writing about the ultimate non-dual nature of reality, eating disorders, stress, disease, or any other subject, he offers the invitation to look at things differently, leaving behind the old, out-grown, painful limitations we have used to bind ourselves in suffering. And then, he welcomes you home to the effortless simplicity of yourself as you are.

Not sure where to begin? Pick up a copy of Lott's most popular book, *You're Trying Too Hard*, which strips away all the concepts that keep us searching for a greater, more spiritual, more peaceful life or self.